COMPLETE ANTI-CANDIDA DIET RECIPES COOKBOOK

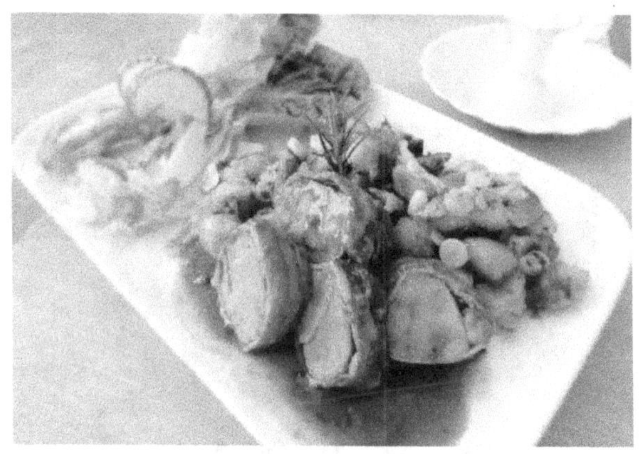

DR. JESSICA SMITH

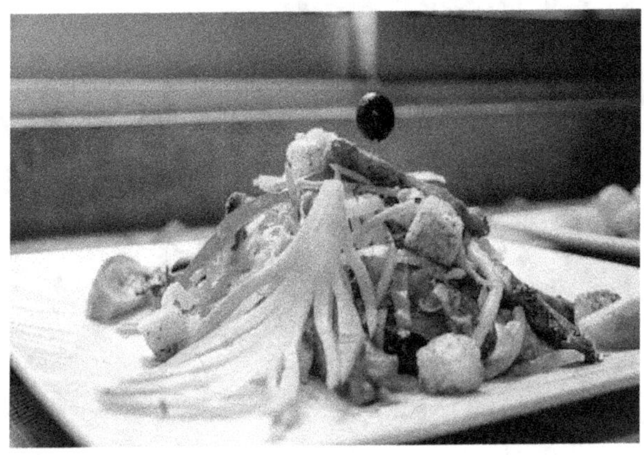

TABLE OF CONTENTS

CHAPTER ONE

How to Use this Cookbook

Using the Complete Anti-Candida Diet Recipes Cookbook can be a straightforward and empowering journey toward better health.

Here are 10 easy steps to help you make the most of the cookbook and implement an anti-Candida diet:

Familiarize Yourself with the Cookbook:

Begin by reading the introduction and any informational sections about the anti-Candida diet. Understand the principles, benefits, and foods to include or avoid.

Gather Ingredients:

Take note of the ingredients required for the recipes. Create a shopping list and ensure you have the essential items in your pantry, including anti-Candida-friendly alternatives.

Meal Planning:

Plan your meals for the week. Consider variety and balance to ensure you're getting a range of nutrients. The cookbook may offer sample meal plans or suggestions.

Start with Simple Recipes:

Begin your journey by selecting simple recipes that align with your taste preferences. Look for recipes marked as beginner-friendly or with minimal ingredients.

Experiment with Substitutions:

If you have dietary restrictions or preferences, feel free to experiment with ingredient substitutions. The cookbook may provide guidance on suitable replacements.

Gradual Implementation:

If transitioning to an anti-Candida diet is new for you, consider gradually implementing the recipes into your routine. Start with a few recipes a week and increase as you become more comfortable.

Stay Hydrated:

Hydration is essential. Ensure you're drinking plenty of water throughout the day. Herbal teas and infusions may also be part of your beverage choices.

Monitor Your Body's Response: Pay attention to how your body responds to the diet. Note any changes in energy levels, digestion, or symptoms related to Candida overgrowth. This feedback can guide your dietary adjustments.

Incorporate Probiotics:

Probiotics play a vital role in supporting gut health. If not included in the recipes, consider adding probiotic-rich foods or supplements to your daily routine.

Seek Professional Guidance:

If you have specific health concerns or conditions related to Candida overgrowth, it's advisable to consult with a healthcare professional or a registered dietitian. They can provide personalized advice based on your individual needs.

Understanding Complete Anti-Candida Diet

The Complete Anti-Candida Diet is a nutritional approach designed to address Candidiasis, an overgrowth of the yeast Candida albicans in the body.

This diet aims to eliminate foods that can contribute to yeast overgrowth, promote a healthy balance of gut bacteria, and alleviate symptoms associated with Candida overgrowth.

The diet typically involves avoiding sugar, refined carbohydrates, and yeast-containing foods, as these can feed the Candida yeast.

Additionally, fermented foods, dairy, and certain fruits are restricted to create an environment less conducive to yeast growth.

Proponents of the Complete Anti-Candida Diet claim that it can help reduce symptoms such as fatigue, digestive issues, and skin problems.

To implement this diet successfully, individuals often focus on whole, nutrient-dense foods, including non-starchy vegetables, lean proteins, and healthy fats.

Probiotic-rich foods, such as sauerkraut and kimchi, may also be included to support a healthy balance of gut bacteria.

It's crucial for individuals considering the Complete Anti-Candida Diet to consult with a healthcare professional or nutritionist to ensure they are meeting their nutritional needs while effectively addressing Candida overgrowth.

While some people report improvement in symptoms, scientific evidence supporting the efficacy of this diet for treating Candida overgrowth is limited, and individual responses may vary.

Principles of Complete Anti-Candida Diet

The Complete Anti-Candida Diet is guided by several principles aimed at controlling and reducing Candida overgrowth in the body.

First and foremost, the diet advocates the elimination of sugar and refined carbohydrates, as these substances provide an ideal environment for Candida yeast to thrive.

This includes cutting out not only obvious sources of sugar but also hidden sugars in processed foods.

The diet also restricts the intake of yeast-containing foods and fermented products, which can exacerbate Candida overgrowth.

Grains that contain gluten, such as wheat, are often eliminated due to their potential to contribute to inflammation and disrupt gut health.

To rebalance the gut microbiota, the Complete Anti-Candida Diet emphasizes the consumption of nutrient-dense, non-starchy vegetables, lean proteins, and healthy fats.

Probiotic-rich foods like sauerkraut, kimchi, and yogurt may be included to promote the growth of beneficial bacteria in the digestive system.

Hydration is another essential principle, encouraging individuals to drink plenty of water to support the body's detoxification processes and overall well-being.

Lastly, the diet often incorporates anti-fungal herbs and supplements, such as garlic and oregano oil, believed to have properties that may help combat Candida overgrowth.

It's important for individuals considering this diet to approach it with caution and seek guidance from healthcare professionals or nutritionists to ensure a balanced and sustainable approach to managing Candida-related issues.

Benefits of Complete Anti-Candida Diet

The Complete Anti-Candida Diet is believed to offer several potential benefits for individuals struggling with Candida overgrowth.

One of the primary advantages is the reduction of symptoms associated with Candidiasis, such as fatigue, digestive issues, and skin problems.

By eliminating sugar, refined carbohydrates, and yeast-containing foods, the diet aims to create an environment in which Candida yeast cannot thrive, potentially alleviating these symptoms.

Furthermore, the diet may contribute to improved gut health by promoting a balanced microbiota.

The emphasis on non-starchy vegetables, lean proteins, and healthy fats encourages a nutrient-dense and anti-inflammatory eating pattern, fostering an environment conducive to a healthier gut flora.

Some individuals report weight loss as a secondary benefit of the Complete Anti-Candida Diet, likely attributed to the reduction in processed foods, sugars, and potential inflammation.

Additionally, adherents of the diet may experience increased energy levels and mental clarity, as the removal of Candida-promoting foods is thought to reduce the burden on the body's detoxification systems.

While anecdotal evidence supports these benefits, it's essential to note that scientific research on the efficacy of the Complete Anti-Candida Diet is limited.

As with any dietary approach, consulting with healthcare professionals is crucial to ensure individual needs are met and to address any underlying health concerns.

Tips for Complete Anti-Candida Diet

Embarking on the Complete Anti-Candida Diet requires commitment and strategic planning. Here are some tips to navigate this dietary approach effectively:

Educate Yourself: Understand the principles of the diet, including which foods to avoid and which to include. Familiarize yourself with hidden sources of sugar and yeast in processed foods.

Plan Meals: Plan well-balanced meals that focus on non-starchy vegetables, lean proteins, and healthy fats. Prepare ahead to ensure compliance with the diet's restrictions.

Read Labels: Scrutinize food labels for hidden sugars, artificial additives, and yeast-based ingredients. Opt for whole, unprocessed foods whenever possible.

Stay Hydrated: Drink plenty of water to support detoxification and overall health. Herbal teas, especially those with anti-fungal properties, can be beneficial.

Incorporate Probiotics: Include probiotic-rich foods like sauerkraut, kimchi, and yogurt (if tolerated) to promote a healthy balance of gut bacteria.

Manage Stress: Stress can contribute to Candida overgrowth. Incorporate stress-management techniques such as meditation, yoga, or deep breathing into your routine.

Gradual Transition: If the diet seems overwhelming, consider a gradual transition by slowly eliminating problematic foods. This can help manage potential detox symptoms.

Consult Professionals: Seek guidance from healthcare professionals or nutritionists familiar with the Complete Anti-Candida Diet. They can provide personalized advice and monitor your progress.

Guidelines of Complete Anti-Candida Diet

Following the guidelines of the Complete Anti-Candida Diet involves a strategic and disciplined approach to address Candida overgrowth. Here are key guidelines to navigate this dietary plan effectively:

Eliminate Sugars and Sweeteners: Remove all forms of sugar, including refined sugars, artificial sweeteners, and even natural sweeteners like honey and maple syrup. Candida thrives on sugar, and cutting it out is fundamental.

Avoid High-Carb and Processed Foods: Steer clear of high-carbohydrate foods, especially refined grains and processed foods, as they can contribute to Candida overgrowth. Opt for whole, unprocessed alternatives.

Minimize Yeast and Fermented Foods: Reduce or eliminate foods that contain yeast or are fermented, as these can exacerbate Candida. This includes bread, vinegar, and most alcoholic beverages.

Choose non-starchy Vegetables: Prioritize non-starchy vegetables, which are rich in nutrients and fiber. These promote a healthy balance of gut bacteria and support overall digestive health.

Include Lean Proteins and Healthy Fats: Incorporate lean proteins such as poultry, fish, and tofu, along with healthy fats from sources like avocados, olive oil, and nuts. These help maintain energy levels and satiety.

Integrate Anti-Fungal Foods: Include natural anti-fungal agents like garlic, oregano, and coconut oil in your diet, as they are believed to help combat Candida overgrowth.

Stay Hydrated: Drink plenty of water to support detoxification and maintain overall health. Hydration is crucial during the Candida cleanse process.

Consider Probiotics and Supplements: Introduce probiotic-rich foods and consider supplements like caprylic acid or grapefruit seed extract, which are thought to have anti-fungal properties and support a healthy gut.

Monitor Progress: Regularly assess your symptoms and adjust your diet accordingly. Gradually reintroduce restricted foods to identify any triggers or sensitivities.

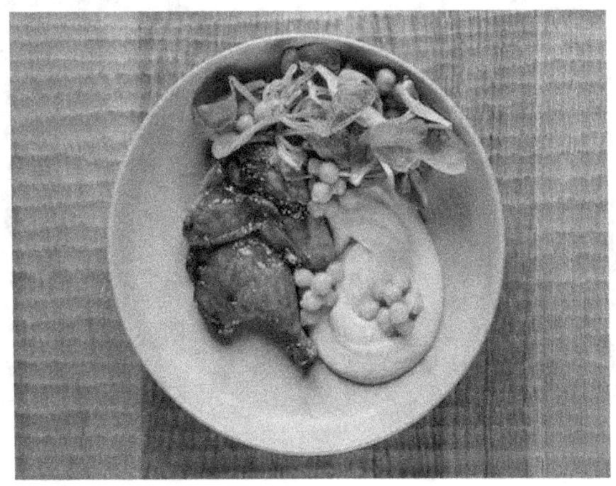

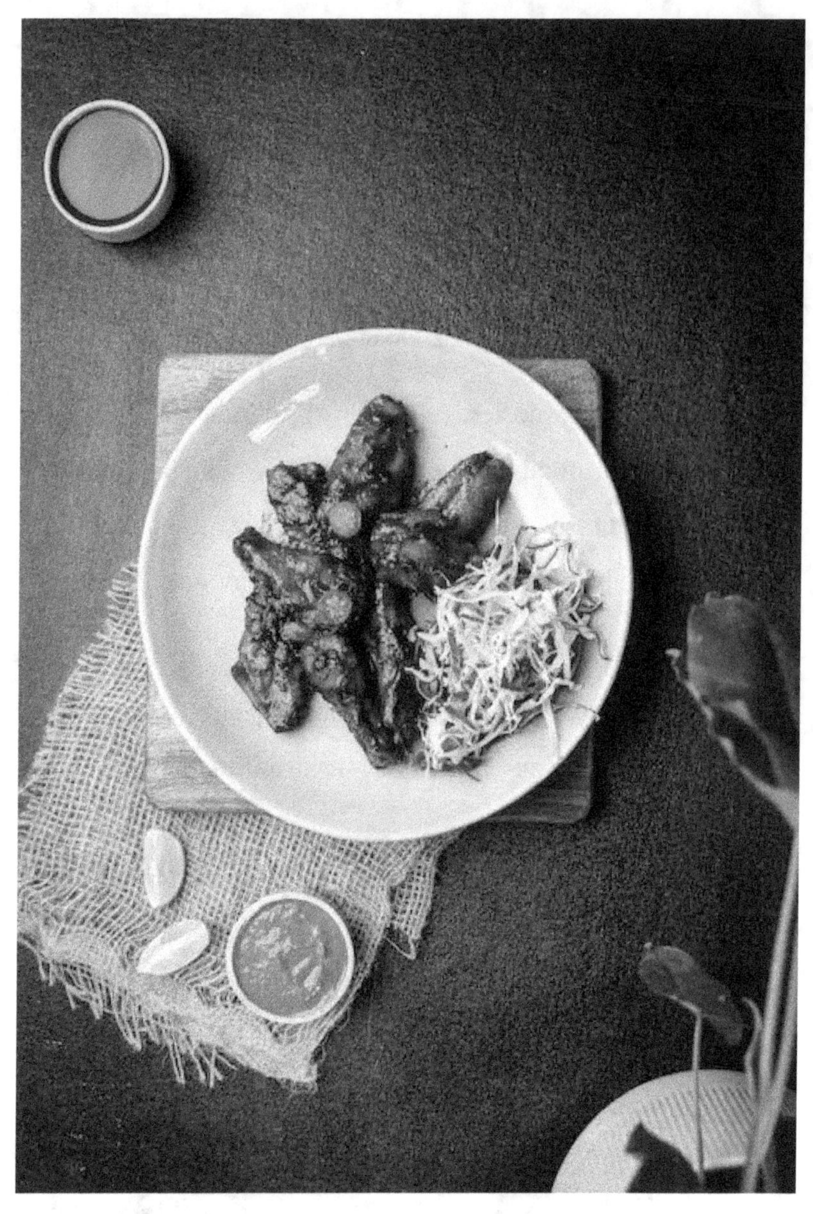

CHAPTER TWO

Complete Anti-Candida Diet Breakfast Recipes

1. Avocado and Turkey Breakfast Bowl

Ingredients:

- 1 ripe avocado
- 100g cooked turkey, shredded
- 1 cup steamed spinach
- 1 tablespoon olive oil
- Salt and pepper to taste

Instructions:

- Mash the avocado and mix it with shredded turkey.
- In a pan, sauté spinach with olive oil until wilted.
- Combine mashed avocado and turkey with sautéed spinach.
- Season with salt and pepper. Serve.

Health Benefits:

- Avocado provides healthy fats and fiber.
- Turkey is a lean protein source.

> ➤ Spinach offers vitamins and minerals.

Preparation Time: 15 minutes

2. Quinoa and Berry Parfait

Ingredients:

- ➤ 1/2 cup cooked quinoa
- ➤ 1/2 cup mixed berries (blueberries, strawberries)
- ➤ 1/2 cup coconut yogurt
- ➤ 1 tablespoon chia seeds
- ➤ 1 teaspoon honey (optional)

Instructions:

- ➤ Layer quinoa, berries, and coconut yogurt in a glass.
- ➤ Sprinkle chia seeds over each layer.
- ➤ Drizzle with honey if desired. Serve chilled.

Health Benefits:

- ➤ Quinoa provides protein and fiber.
- ➤ Berries offer antioxidants.
- ➤ Coconut yogurt supports gut health.

Preparation Time: 10 minutes

3. Smoked Salmon and Cucumber Wraps

Ingredients:

- ➤ 4 cucumber slices
- ➤ 100g smoked salmon
- ➤ 2 tablespoons dairy-free cream cheese
- ➤ Fresh dill for garnish

Instructions:

- ➤ Lay cucumber slices flat.
- ➤ Spread cream cheese on each slice.
- ➤ Place smoked salmon on top.
- ➤ Garnish with fresh dill. Roll up and secure with toothpicks.

Health Benefits:

- ➤ Salmon provides omega-3 fatty acids.
- ➤ Cucumber is hydrating and low in carbs.

Preparation Time: 8 minutes

4. Vegetable Omelette

Ingredients:

- ➤ 3 eggs

- ➢ 1/4 cup diced bell peppers
- ➢ 1/4 cup diced zucchini
- ➢ 1/4 cup cherry tomatoes, halved
- ➢ 1 tablespoon olive oil
- ➢ Salt and pepper to taste

Instructions:

- ➢ Whisk eggs in a bowl.
- ➢ Sauté vegetables in olive oil until tender.
- ➢ Pour whisked eggs over veggies, cook until set.
- ➢ Season with salt and pepper. Fold and serve.

Health Benefits:

- ➢ Eggs provide protein.
- ➢ Vegetables offer vitamins and fiber.

Preparation Time: 12 minutes

5. Coconut Flour Pancakes

Ingredients:

- ➢ 1/4 cup coconut flour
- ➢ 2 eggs
- ➢ 1/2 cup unsweetened almond milk
- ➢ 1/2 teaspoon baking powder

➢ 1/4 teaspoon vanilla extract

Instructions:

➢ Mix all ingredients in a bowl until well combined.

➢ Heat a non-stick pan and ladle batter for each pancake.

➢ Cook until bubbles form, flip, and cook the other side.

➢ Serve with fresh berries.

Health Benefits:

➢ Coconut flour is low-carb.

➢ Almond milk is dairy-free.

Preparation Time: 15 minutes

6. Spinach and Mushroom Scramble

Ingredients:

➢ 3 eggs

➢ 1 cup fresh spinach

➢ 1/2 cup sliced mushrooms

➢ 1 tablespoon coconut oil

➢ Salt and pepper to taste

Instructions:

> ➤ Sauté mushrooms and spinach in coconut oil.
> ➤ Whisk eggs and pour over vegetables.
> ➤ Scramble until eggs are cooked.
> ➤ Season with salt and pepper. Serve warm.

Health Benefits:

> ➤ Spinach is rich in iron.
> ➤ Mushrooms provide antioxidants.

Preparation Time: 10 minutes

7. Chia Seed Pudding

Ingredients:

> ➤ 2 tablespoons chia seeds
> ➤ 1/2 cup unsweetened almond milk
> ➤ 1/4 teaspoon vanilla extract
> ➤ Stevia or monk fruit sweetener to taste
> ➤ Mixed berries for topping

Instructions:

> ➤ Mix chia seeds, almond milk, and vanilla extract.
> ➤ Sweeten to taste and refrigerate overnight.

- ➢ Top with mixed berries before serving.

Health Benefits:

- ➢ Chia seeds are high in fiber and omega-3s.
- ➢ Berries provide antioxidants.

Preparation Time: 5 minutes (plus overnight refrigeration)

8. Almond Butter and Celery Sticks

Ingredients:

- ➢ 2 celery stalks
- ➢ 2 tablespoons almond butter
- ➢ Chia seeds for garnish

Instructions:

- ➢ Spread almond butter on celery sticks.
- ➢ Sprinkle chia seeds for added crunch.

Health Benefits:

- ➢ Almond butter offers healthy fats.
- ➢ Celery is low in carbs and hydrating.

Preparation Time: 5 minutes

9. Turmeric Spiced Cauliflower Rice Bowl

Ingredients:

- ➤ 1 cup cauliflower rice
- ➤ 1/4 teaspoon turmeric
- ➤ 1/4 teaspoon cumin
- ➤ 1 tablespoon olive oil
- ➤ 1/4 cup diced avocado

Instructions:

- ➤ Sauté cauliflower rice in olive oil.
- ➤ Add turmeric and cumin, stir well.
- ➤ Transfer to a bowl and top with diced avocado.

Health Benefits:

- ➤ Cauliflower is low in carbs.
- ➤ Turmeric has anti-inflammatory properties.

Preparation Time: 10 minutes

10. Green Smoothie Bowl

Ingredients:

- ➤ 1 cup spinach
- ➤ 1/2 avocado

- ➤ 1/2 cucumber, peeled

- ➤ 1/2 cup unsweetened coconut milk

- ➤ 1/2 teaspoon spirulina powder

Instructions:

- ➤ Blend all ingredients until smooth.

- ➤ Pour into a bowl and top with chia seeds.

Health Benefits:

- ➤ Spinach provides iron and vitamins.

- ➤ Avocado adds healthy fats.

Preparation Time: 5 minutes

Complete Anti-Candida Diet Lunch Recipes

1. Grilled Chicken and Vegetable Salad

Ingredients:

- ➤ 200g grilled chicken breast

- ➤ Mixed salad greens (lettuce, spinach, arugula)

- ➤ Cherry tomatoes, halved

- ➤ Cucumber, sliced

- ➤ Olive oil and lemon dressing

- ➤ Instructions:

- ➢ Toss salad greens, cherry tomatoes, and cucumber.
- ➢ Top with grilled chicken.
- ➢ Drizzle with olive oil and lemon dressing.

Health Benefits:

- ➢ Chicken provides lean protein.
- ➢ Vegetables offer fiber and vitamins.

Preparation Time: 20 minutes

2. Zucchini Noodles with Pesto

Ingredients:

- ➢ 2 zucchinis, spiralized
- ➢ 2 tablespoons homemade pesto
- ➢ Cherry tomatoes, halved
- ➢ Pine nuts for garnish

Instructions:

- ➢ Spiralize zucchinis into noodles.
- ➢ Toss with pesto and cherry tomatoes.
- ➢ Garnish with pine nuts before serving.

Health Benefits:

- Zucchini is low in carbs.
- Pesto contains anti-fungal garlic.

Preparation Time: 15 minutes

3. Salmon and Avocado Lettuce Wraps

Ingredients:

- 150g grilled salmon
- Large lettuce leaves
- 1 ripe avocado, sliced
- Fresh cilantro for garnish

Instructions:

- Place grilled salmon on lettuce leaves.
- Top with sliced avocado.
- Garnish with fresh cilantro.

Health Benefits:

- Salmon provides omega-3 fatty acids.
- Avocado offers healthy fats.

Preparation Time: 15 minutes

4. Cauliflower Fried Rice with Shrimp

Ingredients:

- ➢ 1 cup cauliflower rice
- ➢ 100g cooked shrimp
- ➢ Mixed vegetables (peas, carrots, bell peppers)
- ➢ 1 tablespoon coconut oil
- ➢ Coconut aminos for seasoning

Instructions:

- ➢ Sauté cauliflower rice and vegetables in coconut oil.
- ➢ Add cooked shrimp and coconut aminos.
- ➢ Stir until heated through.

Health Benefits:

- ➢ Cauliflower is low in carbs.
- ➢ Shrimp provides protein.

Preparation Time: 20 minutes

5. Turkey and Vegetable Stuffed Peppers

Ingredients:

- ➢ 2 bell peppers, halved
- ➢ 200g ground turkey

- ➢ Mixed vegetables (zucchini, tomatoes)

- ➢ 1 tablespoon olive oil

- ➢ Herbs and spices for seasoning

Instructions:

- ➢ Sauté ground turkey and vegetables in olive oil.

- ➢ Season with herbs and spices.

- ➢ Stuff the pepper halves and bake until tender.

Health Benefits:

- ➢ Turkey is a lean protein source.

- ➢ Bell peppers offer vitamins.

Preparation Time: 25 minutes

6. Quinoa Salad with Lemon-Tahini Dressing

Ingredients:

- ➢ 1 cup cooked quinoa

- ➢ Mixed greens (kale, arugula)

- ➢ Cherry tomatoes, halved

- ➢ Cucumber, diced

- ➢ 2 tablespoons lemon-tahini dressing

Instructions:

> ➤ Mix quinoa, mixed greens, tomatoes, and cucumber.
> ➤ Toss with lemon-tahini dressing.

Health Benefits:

> ➤ Quinoa provides protein and fiber.
> ➤ Tahini offers healthy fats.

Preparation Time: 15 minutes

7. Eggplant and Chicken Stir-Fry

Ingredients:

> ➤ 1 cup diced eggplant
> ➤ 150g diced chicken breast
> ➤ Mixed vegetables (broccoli, bell peppers)
> ➤ 1 tablespoon coconut oil
> ➤ Coconut aminos for seasoning

Instructions:

> ➤ Sauté eggplant, chicken, and vegetables in coconut oil.
> ➤ Season with coconut aminos.
> ➤ Stir-fry until cooked through.

Health Benefits:

> - Eggplant is low in carbs.
> - Chicken provides lean protein.

Preparation Time: 20 minutes

8. Cabbage and Turkey Soup

Ingredients:

> - 200g ground turkey
> - 4 cups shredded cabbage
> - 1 can diced tomatoes
> - 1 onion, chopped
> - Vegetable broth
> - Herbs and spices for seasoning

Instructions:

> - Brown turkey and onions in a pot.
> - Add shredded cabbage, diced tomatoes, and broth.
> - Simmer until cabbage is tender.

Health Benefits:

> - Turkey is a lean protein source.
> - Cabbage is low in carbs.

Preparation Time: 30 minutes

9. Sweet Potato and Kale Hash

Ingredients:

- 1 sweet potato, diced
- 1 cup chopped kale
- 1 tablespoon olive oil
- Herbs and spices for seasoning

Instructions:

- Sauté sweet potato and kale in olive oil.
- Season with herbs and spices.
- Cook until sweet potatoes are tender.

Health Benefits:

- Sweet potatoes provide complex carbs.
- Kale is rich in vitamins.

Preparation Time: 25 minutes

10. Shredded Chicken and Avocado Salad

Ingredients:

- 200g shredded chicken breast
- Mixed salad greens (romaine, spinach)

- ➤ Cherry tomatoes, halved
- ➤ 1 ripe avocado, sliced
- ➤ Olive oil and balsamic vinegar dressing

Instructions:

- ➤ Combine shredded chicken, salad greens, tomatoes, and avocado.
- ➤ Drizzle with olive oil and balsamic vinegar.

Health Benefits:

- ➤ Chicken provides protein.
- ➤ Avocado offers healthy fats.

Preparation Time: 20 minutes

Complete Anti-Candida Diet Dinner Recipes

1. Baked Lemon Garlic Herb Chicken

Ingredients:

- ➤ 4 boneless, skinless chicken breasts
- ➤ 2 tablespoons olive oil
- ➤ 2 cloves garlic, minced
- ➤ 1 tablespoon fresh lemon juice
- ➤ Fresh herbs (rosemary, thyme)

➢ Salt and pepper to taste

Instructions:

➢ Preheat the oven to 375°F (190°C).

➢ Place chicken breasts in a baking dish.

➢ Mix olive oil, minced garlic, lemon juice, and herbs.

➢ Coat chicken with the mixture. Season with salt and pepper.

➢ Bake for 25-30 minutes until cooked through.

Health Benefits:

➢ Chicken provides lean protein.

➢ Garlic and herbs have anti-inflammatory properties.

Preparation Time: 35 minutes

2. Cauliflower and Broccoli Alfredo

Ingredients:

➢ 1 cup cauliflower florets

➢ 1 cup broccoli florets

➢ 2 cloves garlic, minced

➢ 1 cup unsweetened almond milk

➢ 2 tablespoons nutritional yeast

➢ Salt and pepper to taste

- ➢ Zucchini noodles or shirataki noodles

Instructions:

- ➢ Steam cauliflower and broccoli until tender.
- ➢ Blend with garlic, almond milk, and nutritional yeast.
- ➢ Season with salt and pepper.
- ➢ Serve over zucchini or shirataki noodles.

Health Benefits:

- ➢ Cauliflower is low in carbs.
- ➢ Almond milk is dairy-free.

Preparation Time: 25 minutes

3. Grilled Salmon with Cilantro Lime Cauliflower Rice

Ingredients:

- ➢ 2 salmon fillets
- ➢ 1 tablespoon olive oil
- ➢ 2 cups cauliflower rice
- ➢ Fresh cilantro, chopped
- ➢ Lime juice

- ➢ Salt and pepper to taste

Instructions:

- ➢ Grill salmon with olive oil, salt, and pepper.
- ➢ Sauté cauliflower rice in olive oil until cooked.
- ➢ Mix in chopped cilantro and lime juice.
- ➢ Serve salmon over cauliflower rice.

Health Benefits:

- ➢ Salmon provides omega-3 fatty acids.
- ➢ Cauliflower is a low-carb alternative.

Preparation Time: 30 minutes

4. Turkey and Vegetable Stir-Fry

Ingredients:

- ➢ 200g ground turkey
- ➢ Mixed vegetables (bell peppers
- ➢ , broccoli, snap peas)
- ➢ 2 tablespoons coconut aminos
- ➢ 1 tablespoon coconut oil
- ➢ Herbs and spices for seasoning
- ➢ Cauliflower rice or quinoa (optional)

Instructions:

> ➢ Brown ground turkey in coconut oil.
> ➢ Add mixed vegetables and cook until tender.
> ➢ Season with coconut aminos, herbs, and spices.
> ➢ Serve over cauliflower rice or quinoa if desired.

Health Benefits:

> ➢ Turkey provides lean protein.
> ➢ Coconut aminos offer a soy-free alternative.

Preparation Time: 20 minutes

5. Eggplant Lasagna

Ingredients:

> ➢ 1 large eggplant, sliced
> ➢ 1 cup ricotta cheese (or dairy-free alternative)
> ➢ 1 cup marinara sauce (sugar-free)
> ➢ 1 cup spinach, chopped
> ➢ 1/2 cup nutritional yeast
> ➢ Herbs and spices for seasoning

Instructions:

> ➢ Roast eggplant slices until tender.

> In a baking dish, layer eggplant, ricotta, spinach, and marinara.

> Repeat layers. Top with nutritional yeast, herbs, and spices.

> Bake at 375°F (190°C) for 30 minutes.

Health Benefits:

> Eggplant is low in carbs.

> Spinach provides vitamins and minerals.

Preparation Time: 40 minutes

6. Shrimp and Zoodles Stir-Fry

Ingredients:

> 200g shrimp, peeled and deveined

> Zucchini noodles (zoodles)

> 1 tablespoon sesame oil

> 2 cloves garlic, minced

> 1 tablespoon coconut aminos

> Sesame seeds for garnish

Instructions:

> Sauté shrimp in sesame oil until cooked.

> Add minced garlic and zoodles.

- ➢ Stir in coconut aminos and cook until zoodles are tender.

- ➢ Garnish with sesame seeds before serving.

Health Benefits:

- ➢ Shrimp provides protein.

- ➢ Zoodles are a low-carb alternative.

Preparation Time: 15 minutes

7. Quinoa Stuffed Bell Peppers

Ingredients:

- ➢ 4 bell peppers, halved

- ➢ 1 cup cooked quinoa

- ➢ 200g lean ground turkey

- ➢ 1 cup diced tomatoes

- ➢ 1/2 cup black beans (optional)

- ➢ Herbs and spices for seasoning

- ➢ Instructions:

- ➢ Preheat the oven to 375°F (190°C).

- ➢ Cook ground turkey and season with herbs.

- ➢ Mix quinoa, turkey, tomatoes, and black beans.

> Stuff bell peppers and bake for 25-30 minutes.

Health Benefits:

> Quinoa provides protein and fiber.
> Bell peppers offer vitamins.

Preparation Time: 40 minutes

8. Avocado and Tuna Salad

Ingredients:

> 2 cans tuna, drained
> 2 ripe avocados, diced
> Cherry tomatoes, halved
> Cucumber, diced
> Olive oil and lemon dressing
> Fresh parsley for garnish

Instructions:

> Combine tuna, diced avocados, tomatoes, and cucumber.
> Drizzle with olive oil and lemon dressing.
> Garnish with fresh parsley.

Health Benefits:

> ➤ Tuna provides protein and omega-3s.
> ➤ Avocado offers healthy fats.

Preparation Time: 15 minutes

9. Coconut Curry Chicken

Ingredients:

> ➤ 4 boneless, skinless chicken thighs
> ➤ 1 cup coconut milk (unsweetened)
> ➤ Curry powder and turmeric
> ➤ Mixed vegetables (broccoli, cauliflower)
> ➤ Coconut oil for cooking
> ➤ Cauliflower rice (optional)

Instructions:

> ➤ Season chicken thighs with curry powder and turmeric.
> ➤ Cook chicken in coconut oil until browned.
> ➤ Add coconut milk and mixed vegetables.
> ➤ Simmer until chicken is cooked through.
> ➤ Serve over cauliflower rice if desired.

Health Benefits:

> Chicken provides protein.

> Coconut milk contains healthy fats.

Preparation Time: 30 minutes

10. Lemon Herb Baked Cod

Ingredients:

> 4 cod fillets

> 2 tablespoons olive oil

> Lemon zest and juice

> Fresh herbs (dill, parsley)

> Garlic powder and onion powder

> Salt and pepper to taste

Instructions:

> Preheat the oven to 400°F (200°C).

> Place cod fillets on a baking sheet.

> Mix olive oil, lemon zest, lemon juice, herbs, and spices.

> Brush the mixture over cod fillets.

> Bake for 15-20 minutes until fish flakes easily.

Health Benefits:

> ➢ Cod is a lean protein source.
> ➢ Lemon and herbs provide flavor without added sugars.

Preparation Time: 25 minutes

Complete Anti-Candida Diet Snacks Recipes

1. Cucumber and Guacamole Bites

Ingredients:

> ➢ Cucumber, sliced
> ➢ 1 ripe avocado
> ➢ Lime juice
> ➢ Salt and pepper to taste

Instructions:

> ➢ Slice cucumber into rounds.
> ➢ Mash avocado and mix with lime juice, salt, and pepper.
> ➢ Spoon guacamole onto cucumber slices.

Health Benefits:

> ➢ Cucumber is hydrating and low in carbs.

> ➢ Avocado provides healthy fats.

Preparation Time: 10 minutes

2. Almond and Coconut Energy Balls

Ingredients:

- ➢ 1 cup almonds
- ➢ 1/2 cup shredded coconut
- ➢ 2 tablespoons coconut oil
- ➢ 1 tablespoon chia seeds
- ➢ 1 tablespoon almond butter

Instructions:

- ➢ Blend almonds in a food processor.
- ➢ Add shredded coconut, coconut oil, chia seeds, and almond butter.
- ➢ Roll into small energy balls.

Health Benefits:

- ➢ Almonds offer protein and healthy fats.
- ➢ Coconut provides medium-chain triglycerides.

Preparation Time: 15 minutes

3. Radish and Hummus Stacks

Ingredients:

- ➤ Radishes, sliced
- ➤ Hummus (sugar-free)
- ➤ Fresh parsley for garnish

Instructions:

- ➤ Spread hummus on radish slices.
- ➤ Stack them and garnish with fresh parsley.

Health Benefits:

- ➤ Radishes are low in carbs.
- ➤ Hummus provides protein.

Preparation Time: 10 minutes

4. Chia Seed Pudding with Berries

Ingredients:

- ➤ 2 tablespoons chia seeds
- ➤ 1/2 cup unsweetened almond milk
- ➤ Mixed berries (strawberries, blueberries)
- ➤ Stevia or monk fruit sweetener (optional)

Instructions:

- ➤ Mix chia seeds and almond milk. Sweeten if desired.
- ➤ Refrigerate overnight.
- ➤ Top with mixed berries before serving.

Health Benefits:

- ➤ Chia seeds are high in fiber and omega-3s.
- ➤ Berries offer antioxidants.

Preparation Time: 5 minutes (plus overnight refrigeration)

5. Turkey and Avocado Lettuce Wraps

Ingredients:

- ➤ Turkey slices
- ➤ Large lettuce leaves
- ➤ 1 ripe avocado, sliced
- ➤ Mustard or sugar-free mayo (optional)

Instructions:

- ➤ Place turkey on lettuce leaves.
- ➤ Top with sliced avocado.
- ➤ Add mustard or mayo if desired.

Health Benefits:

> Turkey provides protein.
> Avocado offers healthy fats.

Preparation Time: 10 minutes

6. Baked Kale Chips

Ingredients:

> Fresh kale, torn into pieces
> Olive oil
> Salt and nutritional yeast (optional)

. Instructions:

> Preheat the oven to 350°F (175°C).
> Toss kale with olive oil, salt, and nutritional yeast.
> Bake for 10-15 minutes until crispy.

Health Benefits:

> Kale is rich in vitamins.
> Olive oil provides healthy fats.

Preparation Time: 15 minutes

7. Avocado and Tuna Lettuce Wraps

Ingredients:

- ➢ 1 can tuna, drained
- ➢ 1 ripe avocado, mashed
- ➢ Lettuce leaves
- ➢ Lemon juice
- ➢ Salt and pepper to taste

Instructions:

- ➢ Mix tuna, mashed avocado, lemon juice, salt, and pepper.
- ➢ Spoon the mixture onto lettuce leaves.

Health Benefits:

- ➢ Tuna provides protein and omega-3s.
- ➢ Avocado offers healthy fats.

Preparation Time: 10 minutes

8. Coconut Yogurt Parfait

Ingredients:

- ➢ Coconut yogurt (unsweetened)
- ➢ 1/4 cup granola (sugar-free)

- ➢ Mixed berries

- ➢ 1 tablespoon unsweetened shredded coconut

Instructions:

- ➢ Layer coconut yogurt, granola, and berries.

- ➢ Top with shredded coconut.

Health Benefits:

- ➢ Coconut yogurt is dairy-free.

- ➢ Berries provide antioxidants.

Preparation Time: 5 minutes

9. Tomato and Basil Bruschetta

Ingredients:

- ➢ Cherry tomatoes, diced

- ➢ Fresh basil, chopped

- ➢ Garlic, minced

- ➢ Olive oil

- ➢ Salt and pepper to taste

- ➢ Cucumber slices (optional)

Instructions:

> Mix tomatoes, basil, garlic, olive oil, salt, and pepper.

> Spoon onto cucumber slices or eat as a salsa.

Health Benefits:

> Tomatoes contain antioxidants.

> Basil offers anti-inflammatory properties.

Preparation Time: 10 minutes

10. Spicy Roasted Chickpeas

Ingredients:

> 1 can chickpeas, drained and rinsed

> 1 tablespoon olive oil

> Paprika, cayenne, and garlic powder

> Salt to taste

Instructions:

> Preheat the oven to 400°F (200°C).

> Toss chickpeas with olive oil and spices.

> Roast for 25-30 minutes until crispy.

Health Benefits:

> Chickpeas provide fiber and protein.

➢ Olive oil offers healthy fats.

Preparation Time: 35 minutes

CONCLUSION

Embarking on the Complete Anti-Candida Diet doesn't mean sacrificing flavor or satisfaction.

This collection of recipes serves as a culinary compass, guiding you through a delicious journey while adhering to the principles of the diet.

From vibrant breakfasts to wholesome lunches and satisfying dinners, each dish is thoughtfully crafted to support your quest for a balanced, anti-Candida lifestyle.

By embracing nutrient-dense ingredients and innovative cooking techniques, these recipes not only aim to combat Candida overgrowth but also promote overall well-being.

Whether you are seeking a nourishing start to your day, a flavorful midday boost, or a comforting evening meal, these recipes offer a diverse array of options that align with the diet's guidelines.

Remember, a holistic approach to health involves not just what we exclude from our diets but also what we choose to include.

These recipes emphasize the power of whole, real foods in creating a positive impact on your digestive health and overall vitality.

As you venture into this culinary exploration, may these recipes inspire creativity in your kitchen and pave the way for a healthier, more vibrant you.

Here's to delicious meals, nourishing choices, and the journey toward a Candida-free lifestyle.

Happy cooking!

www.ingramcontent.com/pod-product-compliance
Lightning Source LLC
Chambersburg PA
CBHW070728260726
48660CB00007B/2776